Beating Alzheimer's Disease for Newly Diagnosed

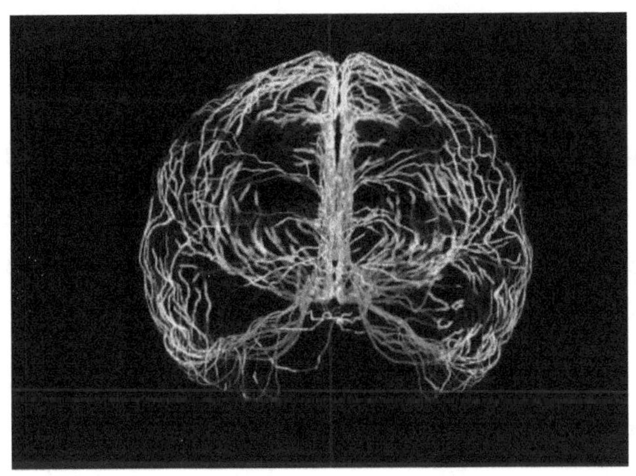

A Step By Step Guide for Seniors To The Diagnosis, Treatment, Management, Medication, And Prevention Of senile dementia.

Rebecca J. Reynolds

Content

INTRODUCTION

Beating Alzheimer's Disease: A Step-By-Step Guide to the Diagnosis, Treatment, Management, Medication, and Prevention of Senile Dementia," we embark on a comprehensive journey into the intricate landscape of one of the most challenging health issues of our time. Alzheimer's disease, a formidable foe that robs individuals of their memories and cognitive abilities, has become a prevalent concern in our aging society. This book seeks to provide not only a profound understanding of the disease but also practical insights and actionable steps for individuals, families, and healthcare professionals alike.

As we navigate the labyrinth of Alzheimer's, we delve into the intricacies of its diagnosis, unraveling the complexities that often shroud early detection. Through the lens of medical advancements and cutting-edge research, we explore the evolving landscape of treatment modalities, dissecting the various approaches that hold promise in mitigating the progression of this formidable condition.

The management of Alzheimer's demands a multidimensional perspective, and this guide meticulously addresses the physical, emotional, and social dimensions of care. From medications that offer a glimmer of hope to innovative therapies that stimulate cognitive function, each facet of the treatment spectrum is scrutinized and presented in a way that empowers individuals and caregivers with informed choices.

Prevention, as the adage goes, is the best medicine. Within these pages, we unravel the intricate web of factors influencing the onset of senile dementia, offering a roadmap for lifestyle modifications that may serve as a shield against its insidious advance. This book is more than a mere guide; it is a beacon of hope, illuminating the path toward understanding, managing, and ultimately triumphing over Alzheimer's disease. Join us as we navigate through the labyrinth, armed with knowledge and compassion, on a mission to beat Alzheimer's and reclaim the essence of a life well-lived.

Myths and Misconceptions about Alzheimer's

Myths and misconceptions surrounding Alzheimer's disease can contribute to misunderstandings and stigmas. It's crucial to address these misconceptions to foster a more accurate understanding of the condition. Here are some common myths along with clarifications:

1. **Memory Loss is a Normal Part of Aging:**
   - Myth: Many believe that forgetfulness is a natural consequence of getting older.
   - Fact: While mild forgetfulness can occur with age, Alzheimer's is not a normal part of aging. It is a progressive neurodegenerative disorder with distinct symptoms beyond typical age-related memory changes.
2. **Only Older People Get Alzheimer's:**
   - Myth: Alzheimer's only affects seniors.
   - Fact: While age is a significant risk factor, early-onset Alzheimer's can occur in people under 65. Younger

individuals, though less common, can also develop the disease.

3. **Alzheimer's is Just Memory Loss:**
   - Myth: Alzheimer's is solely characterized by memory problems.
   - Fact: Alzheimer's can affect various cognitive functions, including language, problem-solving, and judgment. Behavioral changes and mood swings may also occur.

4. **Aluminum Exposure Causes Alzheimer's:**
   - Myth: There's a belief that aluminum from cookware or antiperspirants leads to Alzheimer's.
   - Fact: Scientific evidence does not support a direct link between aluminum exposure and Alzheimer's. The exact cause of Alzheimer's is complex and not fully understood.

5. **Medications Can Cure Alzheimer's:**
   - Myth: Some people think that medications can completely cure Alzheimer's.
   - Fact: While medications can help manage symptoms and slow down the progression of the disease, there is currently no cure for Alzheimer's.

6. **Alzheimer's is Preventable:**

- o Myth: It's commonly thought that certain lifestyle choices can entirely prevent Alzheimer's.
- o Fact: While a healthy lifestyle may reduce the risk, factors like genetics also play a role. Prevention is not guaranteed, but maintaining a healthy lifestyle can contribute to overall well-being.

7. **People with Alzheimer's Can't Understand Anything:**
   - o Myth: There's a misconception that individuals with Alzheimer's are completely unaware and cannot understand their surroundings.
   - o Fact: Cognitive abilities vary among individuals with Alzheimer's. Many can still experience moments of clarity and connection with their surroundings.

8. **Alzheimer's is Just a Memory Problem:**
   - o Myth: Alzheimer's is often oversimplified as a memory disorder.
   - o Fact: It involves complex changes in the brain, impacting multiple cognitive functions. Behavioral and psychological symptoms are also common.

9. **Only Those with a Family History are at Risk:**
   - Myth: Some believe that only individuals with a family history of Alzheimer's are at risk.
   - Fact: While family history increases the risk, sporadic cases also occur. Various genetic and environmental factors contribute to the development of the disease.
10. **Alzheimer's is Contagious:**
    - Myth: There's a misconception that Alzheimer's can be spread through contact with affected individuals.
    - Fact: Alzheimer's is not contagious. It is a non-communicable disease with complex causes rooted in genetics, lifestyle, and other factors.

PART ONE

Understanding Alzheimer's Disease

What is Alzheimer's Disease

Alzheimer's Disease is a progressive neurological disorder that primarily affects memory and cognitive functions. At its core, it involves the accumulation of abnormal protein deposits, called plaques and tangles, in the brain. These formations disrupt communication between nerve cells, leading to the gradual decline of cognitive abilities.

In simpler terms, imagine the brain as a complex communication network. Alzheimer's disrupts this network by creating roadblocks (plaques and tangles), preventing smooth information flow. As a result, individuals may experience memory loss, confusion, difficulty in problem-solving, and changes in behavior.

Over time, Alzheimer's can impact daily life, making it challenging for individuals to perform routine tasks independently. While there's no cure, early detection, support, and certain medications can help manage symptoms and improve the quality of life for those affected. Understanding Alzheimer's as a communication breakdown in the brain can make the concept more accessible to a layperson.

What distinguishes dementia from Alzheimer's disease

The condition of a person's mental abilities is called dementia. It's not a certain illness. It's a mental function decline from a higher level that was severe enough to cause problems in day-to-day functioning.

Dementia patients experience two or more of these particular challenges, such as alterations or reductions in:

- Recollection
- reasoning through and managing difficult jobs.

- Spoken word.
- recognising the link between visual form and space.
- Actions and disposition

The severity of dementia varies. In the least severe level, you can experience a minor deterioration in your mental abilities and need help with everyday chores. In the worst case scenario, a person is totally dependent on other people to assist them with everyday duties.

When illnesses or viruses affect the brain regions responsible for learning, memory, decision-making, or language, dementia results. Approximately two thirds of dementia cases in those 60 years of age and older are caused by Alzheimer's disease, making it the most frequent cause of dementia.

Other typical dementia causes are as follows:

Vascular dementia: Vascular dementia is a common form of dementia. Vascular dementia can affect thinking, memory, language, behavior and personality. Vascular dementia can occur after a stroke or other condition that reduces blood flow to certain parts of the brain. If blood flow is inadequate, necessary oxygen and nutrients are not delivered and brain tissue is damaged. Vascular dementia is diagnosed when at least two types of cognitive decline (such as memory and language) are associated with blockage of blood vessels in the brain and interfere with daily functioning. When fewer than two skills are affected or when cognitive changes do not affect daily functioning, the condition is called severe cognitive impairment. Vascular dementia is the most common cause of senile dementia after Alzheimer's disease.

Dementia with Lewy bodies: Lewy body dementia (LBD) is a type of dementia with Lewy bodies in the brain. Lewy bodies are clumps of protein that accumulate in certain neurons (brain cells). It damages neurons in areas of the brain that affect mental ability, behavior, movement, and sleep.

Dementia with Lewy bodies is a progressive disease in which symptoms begin slowly and worsen over time. LBD is one of the most common causes of dementia in people over the age of 65. The symptoms of LBD can be very similar to other neurological diseases, including Alzheimer's disease and Parkinson's disease. There is no cure for LBD, but the symptoms can be treated with certain medications. You or a loved one may benefit from non-medical treatments such as physical therapy and speech therapy.

Frontotemporal dementia: Frontotemporal dementia belongs to a group of diseases in which the frontal and temporal lobes of the brain deteriorate. As these areas deteriorate, you lose the ability to control them. People with FTD often lose control of their behavior or the ability to speak and understand language.

People with FTD can fall into one of three general clusters of symptoms: Two of these are subtypes of primary progressive aphasia (PPA). PPA is a degenerative brain disease. Despite the name, this is very different from aphasia, a stroke-like condition/symptom that affects the ability to speak and understand language. Three common clusters of symptoms:

- A behavioral variant of FTD (bvFTD).
- Semantic variants in primary progressive aphasia (svPPA).
- Primary progressive nonfluent/verbal aphasia (nfvPPA).

Symptoms associated with FTD can also occur if:

FTD is ALS. When FTD occurs together with amyotrophic lateral sclerosis (ALS).

Parkinson-like FTD syndrome.
Parkinson's disease with progressive supranuclear palsy (PSP) and corticobasal degeneration.

Dementia due to Parkinson's disease:

Parkinson's disease, primarily known for its tremors and movement challenges, can also cast a shadow on the mind, manifesting as dementia. While this aspect can be less talked about, understanding its complexities empowers both patients and their loved ones to navigate this journey with clarity and support.

Imagine the brain as a bustling city square:
Neurons, like citizens, exchange information, relaying messages that keep things running smoothly. In Parkinson's, a protein called alpha-synuclein disrupts this flow, causing tremors

and movement difficulties. This disruption can also spill over into neighboring areas, impacting the cognitive centers and leading to dementia.

The many faces of dementia in Parkinson's:

Mild Cognitive Impairment (MCI): This early stage brings subtle changes in memory, attention, and problem-solving.Misplacing keys, struggling with complex tasks, or forgetting recent events become more frequent.

Parkinson's Disease Dementia (PDD): In this stage, cognitive decline becomes more pronounced, impacting memory,executive functioning, and language.Difficulties with planning, organizing, and communicating become apparent.

Lewy Body Dementia (LBD): This dementia subtype, sometimes associated with Parkinson's, involves widespread alpha-synuclein build-up, leading to additional challenges with visual hallucinations, fluctuations in alertness,and sleep disturbances.

Could Alzheimer's be inherited

Researchers are uncertain about the reasons behind the occurrence of Alzheimer's disease in some individuals while others remain unaffected. However, they have identified various factors that elevate the risk of developing Alzheimer's, with genetic elements being one of them.

Possessing a variant of the apolipoprotein E (APOE) gene heightens the risk, particularly the APOE ε4 variant, which not only increases susceptibility to Alzheimer's but is also linked to an earlier onset of the disease. It's important to note that having the APOE ε4 variant doesn't guarantee the development of Alzheimer's, as some individuals without this variant may still develop the condition.

If an individual has a first-degree relative, such as a biological parent or sibling, with Alzheimer's disease, their risk of developing the condition rises by 10% to 30%. Additionally, individuals with two or more siblings affected by late-onset Alzheimer's disease are three times more likely to develop the condition compared to the general population.

Furthermore, the presence of trisomy 21 (Down syndrome) also amplifies the risk of early-onset Alzheimer's.

Who is impacted by Alzheimer's disease

People over 60 are primarily affected by Alzheimer's disease. The likelihood of developing Alzheimer's disease increases with age beyond 60.

Alzheimer's disease can strike anyone younger than 60; most often, it strikes in their 40s or 50s. This type of Alzheimer's disease is known as early-onset. It is not common. Approximately 10% of AD patients have an early beginning.

What phases does Alzheimer's illness go through

Alzheimer's illness associations and medical care suppliers utilize different terms to depict the phases of Alzheimer's sickness in view of side effects.

While the terms fluctuate, the stages all follow a similar example — Promotion side effects continuously demolish over the long run.

However, no two individuals experience Promotion similarly. Every individual with Alzheimer's infection will advance through the stages at various rates. Not all changes will happen in every individual. It can here and there be challenging for suppliers to put an individual with Promotion in a particular stage as stages might cover.

A few associations and suppliers outline the phases of Alzheimer's sickness regarding dementia:

- prior to clinical Alzheimer's condition.
- Dementia-related mild cognitive impairment (MCI).
- mild Alzheimer's disease-related dementia.

- moderate Alzheimer's disease-related dementia
- severe Alzheimer's disease-related dementia.

The steps are more widely described by other organizations and suppliers as follows:

- Very mild
- moderate

OR

- severe,
- early,
- middle, or late.

Never be scared to ask your loved one's doctor or yourself what they mean when they refer to the phases of Alzheimer's disease using specific terminology.

Preclinical Alzheimer's disease: What is it

Suppliers ordinarily just reference the preclinical stage in research on Alzheimer's sickness.

Individuals with Promotion in the preclinical stage regularly have no side effects (are asymptomatic).

Be that as it may, changes are occurring in their mind. This stage can keep going for quite a long time or even many years. Individuals in this stage aren't generally determined to have Alzheimer's yet in light of the fact that they're working at an undeniable level.

Before symptoms appear, there are now brain imaging tests that can detect deposits of a protein called amyloid in your brain. Amyloid blocks your brain's communication system.

Preclinical Alzheimer's disease: What is it

Healthcare professionals frequently classify memory issues as mild cognitive impairment (MCI) when they become apparent. When compared to other people of the same age, it represents a slight decline in mental abilities.

You might see a minor decrease in capacities in the event that you're in the beginning phases of Alzheimer's. Others near you might see these progressions and point them out. However, the progressions aren't sufficiently extreme to obstruct day to day existence and exercises.

Mild cognitive impairment can result from the effects of a disease or illness that can be treated. However, it is a turning point on the path to dementia for the majority of MCI patients.

Scientists believe MCI to be the stage between the psychological changes found in typical maturing and beginning phase dementia. Different infections can cause MCI, including Alzheimer's or alternately Parkinson's sickness. Essentially, dementia can have different causes.

Risk Factors and Early Warning Signs

Alzheimer's disease is triggered by an abnormal accumulation of proteins within the brain. These proteins, namely amyloid protein and tau protein, lead to the demise of brain cells. The human brain, housing more than 100 billion nerve cells and other cells, collaborates to facilitate crucial functions like thinking, learning, remembering, and planning.

Researchers propose that amyloid protein accumulates in brain cells, forming plaques of increased size. Simultaneously, another protein, tau, intertwines to create tangles. The formation of these plaques and tangles obstructs communication between nerve cells, impeding their ability to execute vital processes.

The gradual death of nerve cells manifests the symptoms of Alzheimer's disease. The initial decline typically begins in a specific region of the brain, often the hippocampus responsible for memory control, and subsequently spreads to other areas.

Despite extensive research, the precise cause of the protein buildup remains elusive to scientists. There is a suggestion that a genetic mutation might instigate early-onset Alzheimer's. Late-onset Alzheimer's, on the other hand, is believed to result from a intricate sequence of brain changes occurring over an extended period. A combination of genetic, environmental, and lifestyle factors likely contributes to the overall causation.

The indications and manifestations of Alzheimer's disease (AD) differ depending on the stage of the condition. Generally, the symptoms of AD encompass a gradual deterioration in one, several, or all of the following:

1. Memory.
2. Reasoning and performance of intricate tasks.
3. Language.
4. Comprehension of visual form and spatial relationships.

5. Behavior and personality.

Individuals with memory loss or other Alzheimer's-related signs might struggle to acknowledge their cognitive decline. These indications may be more apparent to those close to them. Anyone facing symptoms resembling dementia should promptly seek the advice of a healthcare professional.

signs and symptoms of Alzheimer's disease in its mild stage

The initial signs of Alzheimer's disease become apparent during its mild stage. The primary early indication is the inability to remember recently acquired information, particularly regarding recent events, locations, and names.

Additional manifestations of mild Alzheimer's encompass:

- Struggling to articulate thoughts and find appropriate words.

- Experiencing a higher frequency of losing or misplacing objects.

- Encountering challenges in making plans or organizing tasks.

- Facing difficulties in problem-solving.

- Taking an extended time to accomplish routine daily activities.

Individuals in the mild stage of Alzheimer's disease typically retain the ability to recognize familiar faces and navigate to well-known places without significant difficulty.

signs and symptoms of Alzheimer's disease in its moderate stage

The intermediate stage of Alzheimer's, known as Moderate Alzheimer's, is typically the lengthiest phase and can persist for several years. Individuals in this stage often require care and assistance. During this phase, individuals may:

- Encounter heightened memory loss and confusion, frequently forgetting events or details about their lives, such as their phone number or where they attended school.

- Experience growing confusion regarding the day of the week, the current season, and their location.

- Exhibit poor short-term memory.

- Encounter some difficulty recognizing friends and family.

- Repeat stories, thoughts, or events that occupy their minds.

- Struggle with basic mathematical tasks.

- Need assistance with self-care activities like bathing, grooming, showering, and using the bathroom.

- Undergo more pronounced personality changes, displaying agitation or acting out. As the disease advances, they may exhibit signs of depression, apathy, or anxiety.

- Develop unfounded suspicions about family, friends, and caregivers, often referred to as delusions.

- Experience urinary incontinence and/or fecal (bowel) incontinence.

- Encounter disruptions in their sleep patterns.

- Initiate wandering away from their living area.

signs of Alzheimer's disease in its extreme stages

During the advanced phase of Alzheimer's disease, individuals experience profound dementia symptoms and require comprehensive care. Characteristics of this stage include near-total memory loss, a lack of awareness of their surroundings, dependency on assistance for basic daily activities like eating and mobility, a significant decline in communication abilities, and an increased susceptibility to infections, particularly pneumonia and skin infections. Considering the severity of the condition, hospice care may be deemed appropriate during this period to provide comfort and support.

PART TWO

Navigating the Diagnosis

How does one diagnose Alzheimer's disease

Healthcare professionals employ various methods to determine whether an individual experiencing memory issues has Alzheimer's disease. This is crucial as numerous other conditions, particularly neurological ones, can manifest as dementia and mimic Alzheimer's symptoms.

During the initial stages of an Alzheimer's diagnosis, a healthcare provider will inquire about your health, daily activities, and medications. They may also seek input from someone close to you, like a family member, to gain insight into your symptoms. The assessment covers overall health, medical history, ability to perform daily tasks, and changes in mood, behavior, and personality.

Additionally, the provider conducts a physical and neurological exam, a mental status exam evaluating memory, problem-solving, attention, basic math, and language skills. Standard medical tests, including blood and urine tests, are ordered to eliminate other potential causes. Brain imaging tests, such as CT, MRI, or positron emission tomography, may also be performed to support or rule out Alzheimer's disease and other conditions.

Cognitive Tests and Imaging Evaluations

When navigating the complexities of Alzheimer's disease, cognitive tests and imaging evaluations become crucial tools. They act like maps and flashlights, helping doctors illuminate the landscape of your brain and chart a course for diagnosis and management. But for someone unfamiliar with these tools, the process can feel daunting.

Let's shed some light on these assessments and empower you to understand their role.

Cognitive Tests: Imagine your brain as a bustling marketplace, buzzing with neurons bartering information. Cognitive tests are like asking vendors questions to assess their ability to perform their tasks. Here are some common ones:

Mini-Mental State Examination (MMSE): This quick test screens for overall cognitive function, assessing orientation, memory, attention, and language skills.

Montreal Cognitive Assessment (MoCA): This more detailed test evaluates various cognitive domains, including memory, visuospatial skills, executive function, and attention.

Clock Drawing Test: This simple evaluation assesses visuospatial skills and executive function by asking you to draw a clock face and hands at a specific time.

Imaging Evaluations: Think of these as specialized cameras peering into your brain, revealing its structure and activity. Here are two main types:

Computed Tomography (CT) Scan: This scan provides a detailed picture of your brain structure, helping rule out other conditions like stroke or tumors.

Positron Emission Tomography (PET) Scan: This scan measures brain activity, revealing patterns associated with Alzheimer's, such as decreased activity in certain areas.

Note

These tests and evaluations are not definitive diagnoses on their own. Doctors consider them alongside your medical history, symptoms, and physical examination.

Cognitive tests can't pinpoint the exact cause of memory problems, but they can show patterns suggestive of Alzheimer's or other conditions.

Imaging scans can't definitively diagnose Alzheimer's, but they can rule out other causes and provide valuable information about the stage of the disease.

Understanding Test Results and Receiving a Diagnosis

Receiving a diagnosis of Alzheimer's disease can be overwhelming, filled with unfamiliar terms and complex test results. But fear not! Navigating this maze is possible with clear explanations and a supportive approach. Let's break down the process, step-by-step:

The Path to Diagnosis:

Initial Evaluation: Your doctor will likely start by discussing your medical history,symptoms, and concerns. They may also conduct a physical and neurological exam to assess your cognitive abilities.

Cognitive Assessments: Standardized tests, like the Mini-Mental State Examination (MMSE), evaluate memory,attention, language, and problem-solving skills. These tests offer a snapshot of your cognitive functioning.

Imaging Tests: Brain scans, like CT scans or MRIs, rule out other causes of memory problems, such as strokes or tumors. In some cases, PET scans can help detect specific patterns associated with Alzheimer's.

Lumbar Puncture (Optional): In some situations, a spinal tap to analyze cerebrospinal fluid (CSF) may be considered. This fluid bathes the brain and spinal cord, and changes in protein levels can suggest Alzheimer's.

Understanding Your Results:

Test results won't provide a definitive yes or no answer. Instead, they paint a picture of your cognitive strengths and weaknesses, helping your doctor reach a diagnosis based on established criteria.

Cognitive Assessment Scores: Lower scores may indicate potential cognitive decline, but they need to be interpreted in the context of your age, education, and cultural background.

Brain Scans: Abnormalities like shrinkage in specific brain regions can support an Alzheimer's diagnosis, but other conditions can cause similar findings.

CSF Analysis: Elevated levels of certain proteins, like tau and amyloid-beta, can increase the likelihood of Alzheimer's, but these markers aren't foolproof.

Receiving the Diagnosis:

Your doctor will carefully explain the findings, discuss the diagnosis, and answer any questions you have. Remember:

- Diagnosis is not a death sentence. Many people with Alzheimer's live fulfilling lives for years after diagnosis.
- There are different stages of Alzheimer's.Early diagnosis allows for early intervention and management strategies.
- Treatment options and support resources are available. You're not alone in this journey.

Communicating with Loved Ones and Building Support

Alzheimer's disease, with its relentless erosion of memory and communication, can leave loved ones feeling lost and unsure how to connect. But remember, the human spirit is resilient, and even in the face of this challenge, meaningful communication and strong support systems can make a world of difference.

Imagine the brain as a bustling cityscape: Familiar landmarks (memories) stand tall, interconnected by pathways (communication). In Alzheimer's, the fog rolls in, obscuring some landmarks and blurring the paths. Our job is to navigate this new landscape, finding new ways to connect and build bridges of understanding.

Tips for Effective Communication:

Speak slowly and clearly: Use short sentences and simple language, avoiding complex explanations or jargon.

Focus on non-verbal communication: Make eye contact, smile, and use gentle touch to convey warmth and affection.

Listen patiently: Give your loved one time to process information and respond. Don't interrupt or correct them.

Validate their feelings: Acknowledge their emotions, even if you don't understand them. Phrases like "It's okay to feel frustrated" can be helpful.

Focus on the present: Talk about familiar topics, reminisce about shared experiences, or engage in simple activities like listening to music together.

Use humor and playfulness: Laughter can be a powerful tool for connection and emotional release.

Be patient and flexible: Communication will likely require adaptations as the disease progresses. Be prepared to adjust your approach based on your loved one's responses.

Building a Support System:

Talk to your family and friends: Share your concerns and ask for help with caregiving tasks. Don't be afraid to delegate and accept offers of support.

Connect with support groups: Joining a group can provide valuable information,emotional support, and a sense of community. Sharing experiences with others facing similar challenges can be incredibly helpful.

Seek professional help: Therapists and social workers can offer guidance on communication strategies, coping mechanisms, and managing caregiver stress.

Note:

- Communication in Alzheimer's is a two-way street. Be patient, understanding, and willing to adapt your approach.
- Focus on building emotional connections,even if verbal communication becomes challenging.

- Don't hesitate to seek support from family,friends, and professionals. You are not alone on this journey.
- Celebrate small victories: Every moment of connection, laughter, and shared joy is a victory in the face of this disease.

PART THREE

Treatment Options and Management Strategies

Medications and Their Role in Managing Symptoms

Alzheimer's can cause confusion and disorientation in both patients and carers due to its memory loss and twisted mental connections. But in the mist, drugs show up as useful resources—not panaceas, but allies in symptom management and enhanced quality of life. Let's discuss these medications and how they affect people with Alzheimer's disease.

Imagine the brain as a bustling marketplace: Neurons, like vendors, exchange messages using chemical messengers called neurotransmitters. In Alzheimer's, two key neurotransmitters – acetylcholine and glutamate – get disrupted, leading to symptoms like memory loss, confusion, and difficulty thinking.

The two main types of Alzheimer's medications:

Acetylcholinesterase Inhibitors (AChEIs): These act like traffic cops, regulating the levels of acetylcholine. Donepezil (Aricept), Rivastigmine (Exelon), and Galantamine (Razadyne) are some common examples. They can help improve memory, attention, and thinking abilities in the mild to moderate stages of the disease.

Memantine (Namenda): This medication targets glutamate, helping regulate its activity and potentially slowing down the progression of some symptoms, particularly in moderate to severe stages.

Understanding how they work:

1. AChEIs don't cure Alzheimer's, but they can be like fertilizer for the acetylcholine

"vendors," boosting their ability to communicate and potentially improving some cognitive functions.
2. Memantine acts like a security guard, regulating glutamate activity and preventing it from overwhelming the marketplace of neurons, potentially slowing down the progression of certain symptoms.

Important things to remember:

1. Medications don't work for everyone and may have side effects like nausea, vomiting, or fatigue. Talk to your doctor about potential benefits and risks.
2. Medication is just one piece of the puzzle. A healthy lifestyle, including diet, exercise, and mental stimulation, can also play a significant role in managing symptoms.
3. Medications don't stop the disease's progression, but they can offer valuable support in maintaining independence, improving quality of life, and potentially slowing down the decline of some cognitive functions.
4. New medications and treatment approaches are being researched constantly, offering hope for the future.

Non-Drug Therapies: Cognitive Training, Lifestyle Changes

While medications play a role in managing Alzheimer's symptoms, they're not the only weapons in our arsenal. Non-drug therapies, like cognitive training and lifestyle changes, can be powerful allies in the fight to maintain brain health, support cognitive function, and improve quality of life for individuals living with Alzheimer's.

Think of your brain as a garden:

Just like plants need sunlight, water, and care to thrive, our brains benefit from regular stimulation and healthy habits. Non-drug therapies are like nurturing activities that nourish the cognitive soil and help brain cells flourish.

Let's explore some key non-drug approaches:

Cognitive Training:

Brain games and puzzles: Crossword puzzles, Sudoku, and memory games can help stimulate problem-solving skills,attention, and memory.

Learning new things: Taking a class,learning a new language, or playing a musical instrument can challenge the brain in new ways and promote cognitive flexibility.

Computer-based cognitive training programs: Specialized software can provide targeted exercises to improve memory, attention, and other cognitive functions.

Lifestyle Changes:

Physical exercise: Regular physical activity, even moderate-intensity walks,can improve blood flow to the brain,promote neurogenesis (the growth of new brain cells), and boost cognitive function.

Healthy diet: A diet rich in fruits,vegetables, whole grains, and omega-3 fatty acids can nourish the brain and potentially reduce inflammation, which is linked to Alzheimer's progression.

Quality sleep: Aim for 7-8 hours of restful sleep each night. Good sleep is essential for memory consolidation, learning, and overall brain health.

Social engagement: Staying connected with loved ones, participating in social activities, and avoiding isolation can stimulate the brain and provide emotional support.

Stress management: Chronic stress can harm brain health. Techniques like meditation, yoga, and deep breathing can help manage stress and promote relaxation.

Managing Challenging Behaviors and Daily Activities

Living with or caring for someone who exhibits challenging behaviors can be a demanding task. These behaviors can disrupt daily routines, strain relationships, and create feelings of frustration and helplessness. However, with the right approach and understanding, it's possible to manage these challenges and create a more harmonious environment for everyone involved.

Understanding the Why:

The first step in effectively managing challenging behaviors is to understand the underlying cause. Consider the following:

Triggers: What situations or events seem to trigger the challenging behavior?Identifying these triggers can help you anticipate and avoid them, or develop strategies for coping with them.

Communication: Does the person have difficulty communicating their needs or wants? This can lead to frustration and behavioral outbursts. Consider alternative communication methods like picture cards or sign language.

Sensory sensitivities: Does the person have sensory sensitivities that can be overwhelming? Bright lights, loud noises,or certain textures can trigger challenging behaviors. Creating a calming sensory environment can be helpful.

Underlying conditions: Are there any medical or psychological conditions that may be contributing to the behaviors?Consulting a healthcare professional can help identify and address any underlying issues.

Developing Positive Strategies:

Once you understand the underlying cause, you can develop positive strategies to manage the challenging behaviors. Here are some general tips:

Positive reinforcement: Focus on praising and rewarding desired behaviors. This will encourage the person to repeat those behaviors.

Routine and structure: Create a predictable daily routine with clear expectations. This can provide a sense of security and reduce anxiety.

Visual aids: Use visual schedules, charts,or pictures to help the person understand expectations and transitions.

Choice and control: Offer choices whenever possible to give the person a sense of control and autonomy.

Stay calm: It's important to remain calm and patient, even when faced with challenging behavior. Getting upset will only escalate the situation.

Redirection: If a challenging behavior starts, try to redirect the person's attention to a more appropriate activity.

Positive communication: Use clear,concise, and positive language when communicating with the person. Avoid negative phrasing and criticism.

Seek support: Don't be afraid to ask for help from professionals, support groups,or family and friends.

Additional Tips for Specific Situations:

Tantrums: Provide a safe space for the person to calm down and avoid giving in to their demands.

Aggression: Remove yourself or the person from the situation if there is a risk of harm. De-escalate the situation by speaking calmly and avoiding physical contact.

Self-injurious behavior: Seek professional help immediately if the person is engaging in self-injurious behavior.

30 DAYS MEAL PLAN.

Living with Alzheimer's shouldn't limit your culinary adventures! This 30-day meal plan offers tasty, easy-to-digest dishes packed with essential nutrients to support your well-being. Remember, consult a registered dietitian or healthcare professional for personalized dietary recommendations.

Week 1:

Breakfast (Day 1): Scrambled Eggs with Spinach and Cheese: Whisk eggs with milk,sauté spinach, then scramble with feta cheese for a protein-rich start.

Lunch (Day 1): Tuna Salad Sandwich on Whole Wheat Bread: Mix tuna with chopped celery, red onion, and mayonnaise on toasted whole wheat bread for a filling lunch.

Dinner (Day 1): Baked Salmon with Roasted Vegetables: Season salmon with herbs and bake, roast broccoli and carrots for colorful nutrients.

Week 2:

Breakfast (Day 2): Yogurt Parfait with Berries and Oats: Layer Greek yogurt with granola, fresh berries, and a drizzle of honey for a sweet and crunchy treat.

Lunch (Day 2): Chicken Noodle Soup with Vegetables: Simmer chicken, carrots,celery, noodles in broth for a warm and comforting lunch.

Dinner (Day 2): One-Pan Chicken and Veggies: Toss chicken breasts, potatoes,green beans, and olive oil with herbs, roast on a single pan for easy cleanup.

Week 3:

Breakfast (Day 3): Whole Wheat Pancakes with Fruit Compote: Mix whole wheat pancake batter, cook, top with fresh fruit compote for a fiber-rich breakfast.

Lunch (Day 3): Lentil Soup with Whole Wheat Crackers: Make a hearty lentil soup with vegetables and spices, enjoy with toasted crackers for dipping.

Dinner (Day 3): Baked Tilapia with Coconut Rice: Bake tilapia filets, serve with cooked brown rice mixed with coconut milk and chopped pineapple for a tropical twist.

Week 4:

Breakfast (Day 4): Oatmeal with Nuts and Seeds: Cook oatmeal with milk, top with chopped nuts, seeds, and a drizzle of honey for a satisfying morning meal.

Lunch (Day 4): Tuna Melt on Rye Bread:Layer tuna salad with shredded cheese on toasted rye bread for a classic take on lunch.

Dinner (Day 4): Vegetable Fried Rice with Tofu: Stir-fry tofu, chopped vegetables,and cooked rice with soy sauce and spices for a flavorful and healthy dinner.

Note:

- This is just a sample plan, adjust ingredients and portion sizes based on individual needs and preferences.
- Focus on incorporating a variety of colorful fruits, vegetables, whole grains, and lean protein in each meal.
- Choose simple preparation methods like baking, grilling, and steaming for optimal nutrient retention.
- Make the food visually appealing with different colors and textures to stimulate appetite.
- Encourage active participation in meal preparation or setting the table to maintain engagement.

30 DAYS EXERCISE FOR YOU

Staying active, even with Alzheimer's, is key to maintaining physical and mental well-being. This 30-day program offers a variety of safe, enjoyable exercises, tailored to different ability levels. Remember, consult your doctor before starting any new exercise routine.

Week 1: Getting Started

Day 1: Sunshine Stroll: Enjoy a gentle 10-minute walk outdoors, soaking in the sun and fresh air. Listen to calming music or engage in nature observation.

Day 2: Chair Tai Chi: Follow along with a seated Tai Chi video, focusing on mindful movements and deep breathing.

Day 3: Stretching Savvy: Perform gentle stretches for arms, legs, and torso, holding each for 30 seconds. Breathe deeply and listen to your body.

Day 4: Active Fun: Have a dance party! Put on your favorite music and move freely, shaking, swaying, or tapping your feet.

Day 5: Sensory Stroll: Take a 15-minute walk, focusing on sensory experiences. Smell the flowers, touch the leaves, and listen to the sounds around you.

Day 6: Rest and Reflection: Take a well-deserved break. Relax in a comfortable position, focusing on your breathing and peaceful thoughts.

Day 7: Celebrate Success!: Reflect on your achievements this week. Reward yourself with a favorite activity or a delicious treat.

Week 2: Building Momentum

Day 8: Balance Boosters: Stand near a wall for support and raise one leg for 5 seconds, switching legs. Repeat 3 times per side.

Day 9: Chair Cardio: Perform seated leg lifts, raising each leg straight out 10 times. Add arm circles for an extra challenge.

Day 10: Singing Spree: Put on familiar tunes and sing along! Singing is great for memory and mood.

Day 11: Household Hustle: Turn daily chores into exercise. Fold laundry while marching in place, sweep the floor with exaggerated arm movements.

Day 12: Gardening Joy: Spend time in the garden, planting, weeding, or simply enjoying the sights and smells.

Day 13: Relaxation Ritual: Dedicate 15 minutes to deep breathing exercises or guided meditation. Visualization can be calming and beneficial.

Day 14: Socialize and Move: Play gentle games with loved ones, such as throwing a ball or balloon back and forth. Laughter and company boost motivation.

Week 3: Embracing Progress

Day 15: Stair Stepping: Slowly climb and descend stairs 5 times, holding onto the railing for support if needed.

Day 16: Arm Power: Use light weights (soup cans or water bottles) for bicep curls and tricep extensions, 10 repetitions each.

Day 17: Creative Dance: Express yourself through movement! Create your own dance routine or follow choreographed videos aimed at older adults.

Day 18: Neighborhood Explore: Take a longer walk (20-30 minutes) in your neighborhood, exploring new sights and sounds.

Day 19: Sensory Play: Get hands-on with sensory activities like kneading dough, playing with colorful scarves, or sorting textured objects.

Day 20: Mindfulness Moment: Practice mindfulness meditation for 10 minutes, focusing on your breath and bodily sensations without judgment.

Day 21: Celebrate Milestones!: Reflect on your progress and celebrate how far you've come. Reward yourself with a special outing or activity.

Week 4: Maintaining Motivation

Day 22: Partner Power: Ask a friend or family member to join you for walks, chair exercises, or dancing. Social interaction keeps things fun.

Day 23: Balance Beam Walk: Practice walking heel-to-toe along a straight line (imaginary or marked with tape) for improved balance.

Day 24: Music Magic: Create a playlist of uplifting music to motivate you throughout the day. Dance whenever the mood strikes!

Day 25: Household Olympics: Turn routine tasks into mini-challenges. Race against the clock to fold laundry, dust furniture, or vacuum.

Day 26: Nature Connection: Spend time in nature, whether it's a park, your backyard, or even looking out a window. Nature promotes calmness and well-being.

Day 27: Gratitude Practice: Take 5 minutes to reflect on things you're grateful for, focusing on the positive aspects of your life.

Day 28: Celebrate You!: Congratulate yourself on completing this 30-day exercise program! It's an achievement to be proud of, regardless of your ability level or any challenges you encountered along the way. Take some time to reflect on how much you've accomplished and how you feel better physically and mentally. Reward yourself with a special treat, a relaxing activity, or simply spending time with loved ones.

Bonus Week: Keep Moving!

Don't stop moving just because the program is over! Maintain your newfound exercise routine by choosing activities you enjoy and that fit your schedule. Aim for at least 30 minutes of moderate-intensity exercise most days of the week, but remember to listen to your body and take rest days when needed. Here are some ideas to keep you motivated:

- Join a group fitness class designed for older adults. Many communities offer chair yoga, Tai Chi, or low-impact aerobics classes specifically for people with varying abilities.

- Invest in some fitness equipment.Resistance bands, lightweight dumbbells,and balance balls are all great tools for home workouts.
- Find an exercise buddy. Having someone to exercise with can help you stay accountable and make it more fun.
- Track your progress. Keeping a log of your workouts can help you see how far you've come and motivate you to keep going.

Conclusion

In conclusion, navigating the journey of Alzheimer's disease requires a multifaceted approach that prioritizes both quality of life and personal identity for the individual living with it. Maintaining open communication and connection with loved ones is paramount, fostering a sense of belonging and understanding. Building a supportive network, encompassing healthcare professionals, support groups, and advocacy organizations, empowers both the individual and their caregivers. By embracing these strategies, we can illuminate the path forward, ensuring that those living with Alzheimer's continue to experience moments of joy, connection, and a sense of selfhood, even amidst the challenges posed by the disease. Remember, Alzheimer's may dim the memories, but it cannot extinguish the human spirit within. Let us walk alongside our loved ones on this journey, offering unwavering support and cherishing every precious moment together. Together, we can ensure that even in the face of Alzheimer's, the light of a meaningful life continues to shine brightly.

9 7 9 8 8 7 8 2 0 4 9 1 0